# CLINICAL LOGBOOK/PRACTICAL RECORD BOOK

for BSc Nursing Programme

# CLINICAL LOGBOOK/PRACTICAL RECORD BOOK
## for BSc Nursing Programme

*As per the Revised INC Syllabus for BSc Nursing*


**I Clement**
PhD (Nursing) MSc (Nursing) Medical Surgical Nursing
MBA (Education) MSW (Master of Social Work) MA (Sociology) MSc (Physiology) MA (Child Care and Education)
Postgraduate Diploma in Hospital Administration

*Presently*
Professor and Head, Department of Research and Development
RV College of Nursing, Bengaluru, Karnataka, India
*Former,* Professor and Principal
Columbia College of Nursing
VSS College of Nursing, Bengaluru, Karnataka, India
*Professional Assignment*
PhD (N) Guide
INC PhD (N) Guide
Chief Editor for Nursing Journals
Rajiv Gandhi University of Health Sciences
Bengaluru, Karnataka, India
*Professional Life Member*
PhD Society of India, Chennai, Tamil Nadu, India
Nursing Research Society of India, New Delhi, India
Trained Nurses Association of India, New Delhi
Christian Medical Association of India, New Delhi
Indian Society of Psychiatric Nursing, Bengaluru
Medical Surgical Nursing Society of India, Chennai
Indian Society of Neuroscience Nursing, New Delhi
Asian Association of Cardiac Nurses, Kolkata, West Bengal, India
*Health Organization Member*
Indian Red Cross Society, Bengaluru
St Johns Ambulance Association, Bengaluru
General Secretary, Indian Society of Medical Surgical Nurses
*Assignments and Examiner*
Faculty of Nursing, RGUHS, Bengaluru, Karnataka, India
LIC Inspector, Chief Squad, Observer
PhD Research Guide, RGUHS, Bengaluru
UG and PG Examiner, Paper-setter, Valuator other Universities in India
*Professional Activity and Editorial*
MAT Nursing Journal Chief Editor and PUB Journals
Indian Journal of Practical Nursing
National Editorial Advisory Board, New Delhi
Nurses of India (Former) Bengaluru
Chairman-Souvenir Committee, Florence Nightingale Awards-2012
*Winner*
Florence Nightingale Awards-2013
Rajiv Gandhi Education Excellence Award
National Mahila Rattan Gold Medal Award, New Delhi


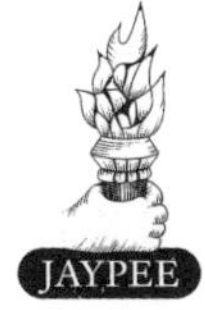



**JAYPEE BROTHERS MEDICAL PUBLISHERS**
*The Health Sciences Publisher*
New Delhi | London

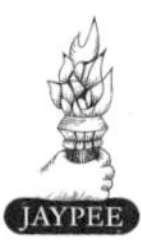

**Jaypee Brothers Medical Publishers (P) Ltd**

**Headquarters**
EMCA House
23/23-B, Ansari Road, Daryaganj
New Delhi - 110 002, India
Landline: +91-11-23272143, +91-11-23272703
+91-11-23282021, +91-11-23245672
E-mail: jaypee@jaypeebrothers.com

**Corporate Office**
4838/24, Ansari Road, Daryaganj
New Delhi - 110 002, India
Phone: +91-11-43574357
Fax: +91-11-43574314
E-mail: jaypee@jaypeebrothers.com

**Overseas Office**
J.P. Medical Ltd
83 Victoria Street, London
SW1H 0HW (UK)
Phone: +44 20 3170 8910
E-mail: info@jpmedpub.com

**EU GPSR** Authorised Representative
Logos Europe, 9 rue Nicolas Poussin
17000, La Rochelle, France
Phone: +33 (0) 6 67 93 73 78
E-mail: contact@logoseurope.eu

Website: www.jaypeebrothers.com
Website: www.jaypeedigital.com



**Inquiries for bulk sales may be solicited at:** jaypee@jaypeebrothers.com

***Clinical Logbook/Practical Record Book for BSc Nursing Programme***

*First Edition*: 2022, **Reprint:** 2025, **2026**

ISBN: 978-93-5465-947-8

*Printed at: Samrat Offset Pvt. Ltd.*

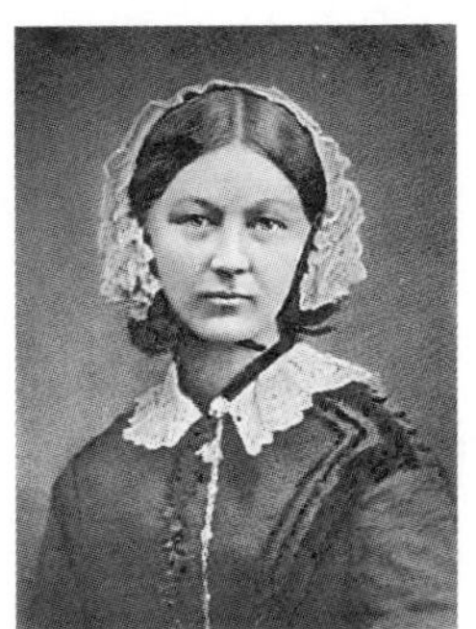

**Florence Nightingale**
**Pioneer of Modern Nursing**

**Born on: 12th May, 1820** **Died on 13th August, 1910**

### “Florence Nightingale Pledge”

*I solemnly pledge myself before God and in the presence of this assembly to pass my life in purity and to practice my profession faithfully.*
*I shall abstain from whatever is deleterious and mischievous, and shall not take or knowingly administer any harmful drug.*
*I shall do all in my power to maintain and elevate the standard of my profession and will hold in confidence all personal matters committed to my keeping and all family affairs coming to my knowledge in the practice of my calling.*
*I shall be loyal to my work and devoted towards the welfare of those committed to my care.*

### “Practical Nurse Pledge”

*Before God and those assembled here, I solemnly pledge;*
*To adhere to the code of ethics of the nursing profession;*
*To co-operate faithfully with the other members of the nursing team and do carryout [sic] faithfully and to the best of my ability the instructions of the physician or the nurse who may be assigned to supervise my work;*
*I will not do anything evil or malicious and I will not knowingly give any harmful drug or assist in malpractice.*
*I will not reveal any confidential information that may come to my knowledge in the course of my work.*
*And I pledge myself to do all in my power to raise the standards and prestige of the practical nursing;*
*May my life be devoted to service and to the high ideals of the nursing profession.*
*Help us spread the word!*

# PREFACE

It gives me immense pleasure to complete this ***Clinical Logbook/Practical Record Book for BSc Nursing Programme*** according to revised syllabus of Indian Nursing Council, New Delhi. Nursing science incorporates clinical competence, critical thinking, communication, teaching learning, professionalism, and caring and cultural competency. Nurses collaborate with other health disciplines to solve individual and community health problems. Nursing facilitates evidence-based practice, compassionate caring among its practitioners in response to emerging issues in health care and new discoveries and technologies in profession. Nursing practice requires personal commitment to professional development and life-long learning. On completion of the clinical practicum, the students will be able to apply nursing process and critical thinking in delivering holistic nursing care.

This record book prepared as per revised INC syllabus which covers all the nursing procedures and provides platform to learn and document the procedures done under the supervision of clinical instructors. I wish all the best to those nursing students who practice their profession by using this book.

**I Clement**

# CONTENTS

# STUDENT PROFILE

Name of the Student: ______________________________ Photo: [ ]

Name of the Institution: ______________________________

Address of the Institution: ______________________________

Name of the University: ______________________________

Reg/Enroll. No.: ______________________________

Date of Birth: ______________________________

Age in Years: ______________________________

Date of Joining to the Institution: ______________________________

Date of Completion: ______________________________

Contact No.: ______________________________

Signature of the Student

Date:

Signature of the Principal

Date:

College Seal

## DECLARATION BY THE STUDENT

I Mr/Ms: ______________________________

S/D/o: ______________________________

Student of: ______________________________

Affiliated to (Name of the College): ______________________________

Name of the University ______________________________

Bearing Enrollment No.: ______________ Seat No.: ______________

Hereby declare that, I have completed all the requirements and procedures mentioned in this clinical log/practical record book within stipulated time limit.

Signature of Student

Date:

Place:

# DECLARATION BY THE PRINCIPAL

Mr/Ms: ______________________________

S/D/o: ______________________________

Student of: ______________________________

Affiliated to (Name of the College): ______________________________

Name of the University: ______________________________

Bearing Enrollment No.: ______________ Seat No.: ______________

Has completed all the requirements and procedures mentioned in this clinical log/practical record book within stipulated time limit (from: ______________ to ______________) for partial fulfillment of requirements for the award of Basic BSc Nursing.

Signature of Principal

Date:

Place:

## DESCRIPTION OF BSC NURSING PROGRAMME

| Sem. | | Subjects |
|---|---|---|
| | | **FIRST YEAR** |
| **I** | | **Semester-I** |
| | 1. | Communicative English |
| | 2. | Applied Anatomy and Physiology |
| | 3. | Applied Sociology and Psychology |
| | 4. | Nursing foundations-I |
| | | **Mandatory module:** First aid (as part of Nursing Foundation-I Course) |
| **II** | | **Semester-II** |
| | 1. | Applied biochemistry |
| | 2. | Applied nutrition and dietetics |
| | 3. | Nursing foundations II |
| | 4. | Health/nursing informatics and technology |
| | | **Mandatory module:** Health assessment (as part of Nursing Foundation-II Course) |
| | | **SECOND YEAR** |
| **III** | | **Semester-III** |
| | 1. | Applied microbiology, and infection control including safety |
| | 2. | Pharmacology I |
| | 3. | Pathology I |
| | 4. | Adult health (medical surgical ) nursing I with integrated pathophysiology |
| | | **Mandatory module:** BCLS (as part of adult health nursing-I) |
| **IV** | | **Semester-IV** |
| | 1. | Pharmacology II |
| | 2. | Pathology II and genetics |
| | 3. | Adult health (medical surgical) nursing II including geriatrics with integrated pathophysiology |
| | 4. | Professionalism, professional values and ethics including bioethics |
| | | **Mandatory module:** Fundaments of prescribing under pharmacology-II, palliative care module under adult health nursing-II |
| | | **THIRD YEAR** |
| **V** | | **Semester-V** |
| | 1. | Child health nursing I |
| | 2. | Mental health nursing I |
| | 3. | Community health nursing (including environmental science and epidemiology) |
| | 4. | Educational/technology/nursing education |
| | 5. | Introduction to forensic nursing and Indian laws |
| | | **Mandatory modules:** Essential Newborn Care (ENBC), Facility based Newborn Care (FBNBC), IMNCI and PLS (as part of child health nursing) |

| Sem. | | Subjects |
|---|---|---|
| **VI** | | **Semester-VI** |
| | 1. | Child health nursing-II |
| | 2. | Mental health nursing-II |
| | 3. | Nursing management and leadership |
| | 4. | Midwifery/obstetrics and gynecology (OBG) nursing-I |
| | | **Mandatory modules:** SBA module under OBG nursing I/II (VI/VII semester) |
| **VII** | | **Semester-VII** |
| | 1. | Community health nursing-II |
| | 2. | Nursing research and statistics |
| | 3. | Midwifery/Obstetrics and Gynecology (OBG) Nursing-II |
| | | Mandatory modules: Safe delivery app under OBG nursing I/II (VI/VII Semester) |
| **VIII** | | **Semester-VIII** |
| | | Internship (intensive practicum/residency posting) |

(Modules both mandatory and elective shall be certified by the institution/external agency)

# COURSE OF INSTRUCTION WITH CREDIT SCORE

Theory: 20 hours-1 credit, Lab Skill: 40 hours-1 credit, Clinical: 80 hours-1 credit

| S. No. | Sem. | Course code | Course/subject | Theory credit | Theory hours | Lab/ skill labs credit | Lab/ skill lab hours | Clinical credit | Clinical hours | Total credit | Total hours |
|---|---|---|---|---|---|---|---|---|---|---|---|
| 1. | First | ENGL101 | Communicative english | 2 | 40 | | | | | | 40 |
| | | ANAT105 | Applied anatomy | 3 | 60 | | | | | | 60 |
| | | PHYS110 | Applied physiology | 3 | 60 | | | | | | 60 |
| | | SOCI115 | Applied sociology | 3 | 60 | | | | | | 60 |
| | | PSYC120 | Applied psychology | 3 | 60 | | | | | | 60 |
| | | N-NF (I)125 | Nursing foundation-I including first aid module | 6 | 120 | 2 | 80 | 2 | 160 | 10 | 360 |
| | | SSCC(I)130 | Self-study/co-curricular | | | | | | | | 40+40 |
| | | | **Total** | 20 | 400 | 2 | 80 | 2 | 160 | 20 + 2 + 2 = 24 | 640 + 80 = 720 |
| 2. | Second | BIOC135 | Applied biochemistry | 2 | 40 | | | | | | 40 |
| | | NUTR140 | Applied nutrition and dietetics | 3 | 60 | | | | | | 60 |
| | | N-NF-II125 | Nursing foundation-II including health assessment module | 6 | 120 | 3 | 120 | 4 | 320 | | 560 |
| | | NHIT145 | Health/nursing informatics and technology | 2 | 40 | 1 | 40 | | | | 80 |
| | | SSCC (II) | Self-study/co-curricular | | | | | | | | 40+20 |
| | | | **Total** | 13 | 260 | 4 | 160 | 4 | 320 | 13 + 4 + 4 = 21 | 740 + 60 = 800 |
| 3. | Third | MICR | Applied microbiology and infection control including safety | 2 | 40 | 1 | 40 | | | | 80 |
| | | PHAR-I-205 | Pharmacology-I | 1 | 20 | | | | | | 20 |
| | | PATH-I-210 | Pathology-I | 1 | 20 | | | | | | 20 |
| | | N-AHN-I-215 | Adult health nursing-I integrated pathophysiology including BCLS module | 7 | 140 | 1 | 40 | 6 | 480 | | 660 |

| S. No. | Sem. | Course code | Course/subject | Theory credit | Theory hours | Lab/ skill labs credit | Lab/ skill lab hours | Clinical credit | Clinical hours | Total credit | Total hours |
|---|---|---|---|---|---|---|---|---|---|---|---|
| | | SSCC (I)220 | Self-study/Co-curricular | | | | | | | | |
| | | | **Total** | 11 | 220 | 2 | 80 | 6 | 480 | 11+2 + 6 =19 | 780 + 20 = 800 |
| 4. | Fourth | PHAR-II-205 | Pharmacology-II including fundaments of prescribing module | 3 | 60 | | | | | | 60 |
| | | PATH-I-210 | Pathology-I and genetics | 1 | 20 | | | | | | 20 |
| | | N-AHN-I-225 | Adult health nursing-II integrated pathophysiology including geriatric nursing +palliative care module | 7 | 140 | 1 | 40 | 6 | 480 | | 660 |
| | | PROF 230 | Professionalism, professional values and ethics including bioethics | 1 | 20 | | | | | | 20 |
| | | SSCC (I)220 | Self-study/co-curricular | | | | | | | | 40 |
| | | | **Total** | 12 | 240 | 1 | 40 | 6 | 480 | 12 + 1 + 6 = 19 | 760 + 40 = 800 |
| 5. | Fifth | N-CHN-I-301 | Child health nursing-I including essential newborn care (ENBC), FBNC, IMNCI and PLS module | 3 | 60 | 1 | 40 | 2 | 80 | | 260 |
| | | N-MHN-I-305 | Mental health nursing-I | 3 | 60 | | | 1 | 160 | | 140 |
| | | N-COM-I-310 | Community health nursing-I including environmental science and epidemiology | 5 | 100 | | | 2 | 160 | | 260 |
| | | EDU215 | Educational technology/ nursing education | 2 | 40 | 1 | 40 | | | | 80 |
| | | N-FORN320 | Introduction to forensic nursing and Indian laws | 1 | 20 | | | | | | 20 |
| | | SSCC (I)325 | Self-study/co-curricular | | | | | | | | 20+20 |
| | | | **Total** | 14 | 280 | 2 | 80 | 5 | 400 | 14 + 2 + 5 = 21 | 760 + 40 = 800 |

| S. No. | Sem. | Course code | Course/subject | Theory credit | Theory hours | Lab/ skill labs credit | Lab/ skill lab hours | Clinical credit | Clinical hours | Total credit | Total hours |
|---|---|---|---|---|---|---|---|---|---|---|---|
| 6. | Sixth | N-CHN-II-301 | Child health nursing-II | 2 | 40 | | | 1 | 80 | | 120 |
| | | N-MHN-II-305 | Mental health nursing-II | 2 | 40 | | | 2 | 160 | | 200 |
| | | NMLE330 | Nursing management and leadership | 3 | 60 | | | 1 | 80 | | 140 |
| | | N-MIDW-I/ OBGN335 | Midwifery/ obstetrics and gynecology (OBG) Nursing-I including SBA module | 3 | 60 | 1 | 40 | 3 | 240 | | 340 |
| | | SSCC (I)325 | Self-study/co-curricular | | | | | | | | |
| | | | **Total** | 10 | 200 | 1 | 40 | 7 | 560 | 10 + 1 + 7 = 18 | 800 |
| 7. | Seventh | N-COMN-II-401 | Community health nursing-II | 5 | 100 | | | 2 | 160 | | 260 |
| | | NRST405 | Nursing research and statistics | 2 | 40 | 2 | 80 (pro-ject - 40) | | | | 120 |
| | | N-MIDW-II/ OBGN 410 | Midwifery/ obstetrics and gynecology (OBG) Nursing-II including safe delivery app module | 3 | 60 | 1 | 40 | 4 | 320 | | 420 |
| | | | **Total** | 10 | 200 | 3 | 120 | 6 | 480 | 10 + 3 + 6 = 19 | 800 |
| 8. | Eight (Intern-ship) | INTE415 | Community health nursing—4 weeks | | | | | | | | |
| | | INTE420 | Adult health nursing—6 weeks | | | | | | | | |
| | | INTE425 | Child health nursing—4 weeks | | | | | | | | |
| | | INTE430 | Mental health nursing—4 weeks | | | | | | | | |
| | | INTE435 | Midwifery—4 weeks | | | | | | | | |
| | | | Total = 22 weeks | | | | | 12 (1 credit = 4 hours per week per seme-ster | | | 1056 (4 hours x 22 weeks = 88 hours x 12 credit = 1056 hours (48 hours per week x 22 weeks) |

# SCHEME OF EXAMINATION

## FIRST SEMESTER

| S. No. | Course | Assessment (Marks) | | | | |
|---|---|---|---|---|---|---|
| | | Internal | End semester exam | End semester University exam | Hours | Total marks |
| **Theory** | | | | | | |
| 1. | Communicative english | 25 | 25 | | 2 | 50 |
| 2. | Applied anatomy and applied physiology | 25 | | 75 | 3 | 100 |
| 3. | Applied sociology and applied psychology | 25 | | 75 | 3 | 100 |
| 4. | *Nursing foundation | *25 | | | | |
| **Practical** | | | | | | |
| 5. | *Nursing foundation | *25 | | | | |

*Will be added to the internal marks of nursing foundation II theory and practical respectively in the next semester (Total weightage remains the same)

## SECOND SEMESTER

| S. No. | Course | Assessment (Marks) | | | | |
|---|---|---|---|---|---|---|
| | | Internal | End semester exam | End semester University exam | Hours | Total marks |
| **Theory** | | | | | | |
| 1. | Applied biochemistry and applied nutrition and dietetics | 25 | | 75 | 3 | 100 |
| 2. | Nursing foundation (I and II) | 25 (Sem-I = 25 + Sem-II=25) Weightage | | 75 | 3 | 100 |
| 3. | Health informatics and technology | 25 | 25 | | | 50 |
| **Practical** | | | | | | |
| 4. | Nursing foundation (I and II) | 50 (Sem-I = 25 + Sem-II = 25) | | 50 | | 100 |

## THIRD SEMESTER

| S. No. | Course | Assessment (Marks) | | | | |
|---|---|---|---|---|---|---|
| | | Internal | End semester exam | End semester University exam | Hours | Total marks |
| **Theory** | | | | | | |
| 1. | Applied microbiology and infection control including safety | 25 | | 75 | 3 | 100 |
| 2. | Pharmacology I and pathology I | *25 | | | | |
| 3. | Adult health nursing I | 25 | | 75 | 3 | 100 |
| **Practical** | | | | | | |
| 4. | Adult health nursing I | 50 | | 50 | | 100 |

*Will be added to the internal marks of pharmacology II and pathology II and genetics in the next semester (Total weightage remains the same)

## FOURTH SEMESTER

| S. No. | Course | Assessment (Marks) | | | | |
|---|---|---|---|---|---|---|
| | | Internal | End semester exam | End semester University exam | Hours | Total marks |
| | | **Theory** | | | | |
| 1. | Pharmacology II and pathology II and genetics | 25 | | 75 | 3 | 100 |
| 2. | Adult health nursing II | 25 | | 75 | 3 | 100 |
| 3. | Professionalism, professional values and ethics including bioethics | 25 | 25 | | 2 | 50 |
| | | **Practical** | | | | |
| 4. | Adult health nursing II | 50 | | 50 | | 100 |

## FIFTH SEMESTER

| S. No. | Course | Assessment (Marks) | | | | |
|---|---|---|---|---|---|---|
| | | Internal | End semester exam | End semester University exam | Hours | Total marks |
| | | **Theory** | | | | |
| 1. | Child health nursing I | *25 | | | | |
| 2. | Mental health nursing I | *25 | | | | |
| 3. | Community health nursing-I including environmental science and epidemiology | 25 | | 75 | 3 | 100 |
| 4. | Educational technology/nursing education | 25 | | 75 | 3 | 100 |
| 5. | Introduction to forensic nursing and Indian laws | 25 | 25 | | | 50 |
| | | **Practical** | | | | |
| 6. | Child health nursing I | *25 | | | | |
| 7. | Mental health nursing I | *25 | | | | |
| 8. | Community health nursing-I | 50 | | 50 | | 100 |

*Will be added to the internal marks of child health nursing II and mental health nursing II in both theory and practical respectively in the next semester (Total weightage remains the same)

## SIXTH SEMESTER

| S. No. | Course | Assessment (Marks) | | | | |
|---|---|---|---|---|---|---|
| | | Internal | End semester exam | End semester University exam | Hours | Total marks |
| | | **Theory** | | | | |
| 1. | Child health nursing I and II | 25 | | 75 | 3 | 100 |
| 2. | Mental health nursing I and II | 25 | | 75 | 3 | 100 |

| S. No. | Course | Assessment (Marks) | | | | |
|---|---|---|---|---|---|---|
| | | Internal | End semester exam | End semester University exam | Hours | Total marks |
| 3. | Nursing management and leadership | 25 | | 75 | 3 | 100 |
| 4. | Midwifery/obstetrics and gynecology-I | *25 | | | | |
| | | Practical | | | | |
| 5. | Child health nursing I and II | 50 | | 50 | | 100 |
| 6. | Mental health nursing I and II | 50 | | 50 | | 100 |
| 7. | Midwifery/obstetrics and gynecology-I | *25 | | | | |

*Will be added to the internal marks of midwifery II theory and practical respectively in the next semester (Total weightage remains the same)

## SEVENTH SEMESTER

| S. No. | Course | Assessment (Marks) | | | | |
|---|---|---|---|---|---|---|
| | | Internal | End semester exam | End semester University exam | Hours | Total marks |
| | | Theory | | | | |
| 1. | Community health nursing II | 25 | | 75 | 3 | 100 |
| 2. | Nursing research and statistics | 25 | | 75 | 3 | 100 |
| 3. | Midwifery/obstetrics (OBG) and gynecology-I and II | 25 | | 75 | 3 | 100 |
| | | Practical | | | | |
| 4. | Community health nursing II | 50 | | 50 | | 100 |
| 5. | Midwifery/obstetrics (OBG) and gynecology-I and II | 50 | | 50 | | 100 |

## EIGHTH SEMESTER

| S. No. | Course | Assessment (Marks) | | | | |
|---|---|---|---|---|---|---|
| | | Internal | End semester exam | End semester University exam | Hours | Total marks |
| | | Practical | | | | |
| 1. | Competency Assessment | 100 | | 100 | | 200 |

## SEMESTER -I: NURSING FOUNDATION-I

| S. No. | Procedural competencies/skill | Performs independently | Assist/observes procedure (A/O) | Date | | Signature of the tutor/ faculty |
|---|---|---|---|---|---|---|
| | | | | Skill lab/simulation lab | Clinical area | |
| **I. Communication and documentation** | | | | | | |
| 1. | Maintain communication and interpersonal relationship with patient and families | | | | | |
| 2. | Verbal report | | | | | |
| 3. | Recording/ documentation of patient care (written report) | | | | | |
| **II. Monitoring vital signs** | | | | | | |
| *A. Temperature* | | | | | | |
| 4. | Oral | | | | | |
| 5. | Axillary | | | | | |
| 6. | Rectal | | | | | |
| 7. | Tympanic | | | | | |
| *B. Pulse* | | | | | | |
| 8. | Radial | | | | | |
| 9. | Apical | | | | | |
| 10. | Respiration | | | | | |
| 11. | Blood pressure | | | | | |
| **III. Hot and cold applications** | | | | | | |
| 12. | Cold compress | | | | | |
| 13. | Hot compress | | | | | |
| 14. | Ice cap | | | | | |
| 15. | Tepid sponge | | | | | |
| **IV. Health assessment (Basic—first year level)** | | | | | | |
| 16. | Health history | | | | | |
| 17. | Physical assessment-general and system wice | | | | | |
| 18. | Documentation of findings | | | | | |
| **V. Infection control in clinical settings** | | | | | | |
| 19. | Hand hygiene (hand washing and hand rub) | | | | | |
| 20. | Use of personal and protective equipment | | | | | |

| S. No. | Procedural competencies/skill | Performs independently | Assist/observes procedure (A/O) | Date | | Signature of the tutor/ faculty |
|---|---|---|---|---|---|---|
| | | | | Skill lab/simulation lab | Clinical area | |
| **VI. Comfort** | | | | | | |
| 21. | Open bed | | | | | |
| 22. | Occupied bed | | | | | |
| 23. | Post-operative bed | | | | | |
| 24. | Supine position | | | | | |
| 25. | Fowler's position | | | | | |
| 26. | Lateral position | | | | | |
| 27. | Prone position | | | | | |
| 28. | Semi-prone position | | | | | |
| 29. | Trendelenburg position | | | | | |
| 30. | Lithotomy position | | | | | |
| 31. | Changing position of helpless patient (moving/turning/ logrolling) | | | | | |
| 32. | Cardiac table/over-bed table | | | | | |
| 33. | Back rest | | | | | |
| 34. | Bed cradle | | | | | |
| 35. | Pain assessment (initial and reassessment) | | | | | |
| **VII. Safety** | | | | | | |
| 36. | Side rail | | | | | |
| 37. | Restraints (physical) | | | | | |
| 38. | Fall risk assessment and post fall assessment | | | | | |
| **VIII. Admission and discharge** | | | | | | |
| 39. | Admission | | | | | |
| 40. | Discharge | | | | | |
| 41. | Transfer (within hospital) | | | | | |
| **IX. Mobility** | | | | | | |
| 42. | Ambulation | | | | | |
| 43. | Transferring patient from and to bed and wheel chair | | | | | |
| 44. | Transferring patient from and to bed and stretcher | | | | | |
| 45. | Range of motion exercises (ROM) | | | | | |

| S. No. | Procedural competencies/skill | Performs independently | Assist/observes procedure (A/O) | Date | | Signature of the tutor/ faculty |
|---|---|---|---|---|---|---|
| | | | | Skill lab/simulation lab | Clinical area | |
| **X. Patient education** | | | | | | |
| 46. | Individual patient teaching | | | | | |

Signature of Class-coordinator

Signature of Principal with seal

**Internal Practical Examination of Nursing Foundation**

Signature of Examiner-I

Signature of Examiner-II

Name:

Name:

Date:

Date:

## SEMESTER -II: NURSING FOUNDATION-II

| S. No. | Procedural competencies/ skill | Performs independently | Assist/observes procedure (A/O) | Date | | Signature of the tutor/ faculty |
|---|---|---|---|---|---|---|
| | | | | Skill lab/ simulation lab | Clinical area | |
| **XI. Hygiene** | | | | | | |
| 47. | Sponge bath | | | | | |
| 48. | Pressure injury assessment | | | | | |
| 49. | Skin care and care of pressure points | | | | | |
| 50. | Oral hygiene | | | | | |
| 51. | Hair wash | | | | | |
| 52. | Pediculosis treatment | | | | | |
| 53. | Perineal care/meatal care | | | | | |
| 54. | Urinary catheter care | | | | | |
| **XII. Nursing process—basic level** | | | | | | |
| 55. | Assessment and formulating nursing diagnosis | | | | | |
| 56. | Planning the nursing care | | | | | |
| 57. | Implementation of care | | | | | |
| 58. | Evaluation of care (reassessment and modification) | | | | | |
| **XIII. Nutrition and fluid balance** | | | | | | |
| 59. | 24 hours dietary recall | | | | | |
| 60. | Planning well balanced diet | | | | | |
| 61. | Making fluid chart | | | | | |
| 62. | Preparation of nasogastric tube feed | | | | | |
| 63. | Nasogastric tube feeding | | | | | |
| 64. | Maintaining intake and output chart | | | | | |
| 65. | Intravenous infusion plan | | | | | |
| **XIV. Elimination** | | | | | | |
| 66. | Providing bed pan | | | | | |
| 67. | Providing urinal | | | | | |
| 68. | Enema | | | | | |
| 69. | Bowel wash | | | | | |

| S. No. | Procedural competencies/ skill | Performs independently | Assist/observes procedure (A/O) | Date | | Signature of the tutor/ faculty |
|---|---|---|---|---|---|---|
| | | | | Skill lab/ simulation lab | Clinical area | |
| **XV. Diagnostic test** | | | | | | |
| *A. Specimen collection* | | | | | | |
| 70. | Urine specimen for routine analysis | | | | | |
| 71. | Urine specimen for culture | | | | | |
| 72. | Timed urine specimen collection | | | | | |
| 73. | Feces specimen for routine | | | | | |
| 74. | Sputum culture | | | | | |
| *B. Urine test* | | | | | | |
| 75. | Ketones | | | | | |
| 76. | Albumin | | | | | |
| 77. | Reaction | | | | | |
| 78. | Specific gravity | | | | | |
| **XVI. Oxygenation needs/promoting respiration** | | | | | | |
| 79. | Deep breathing and coughing exercises | | | | | |
| 80. | Steam inhalation | | | | | |
| 81. | Oxygen administration using face mask | | | | | |
| 82. | Oxygen administration using nasal prongs | | | | | |
| **XVII. Medication administration** | | | | | | |
| 83. | Oral medications | | | | | |
| 84. | Intramuscular | | | | | |
| 85. | Subcutaneous | | | | | |
| 86. | Rectal suppositories | | | | | |
| **XVIII. Death and dying** | | | | | | |
| 87. | Death care/last office | | | | | |
| **XIX. First aid and emergencies** | | | | | | |
| | Bandages and binders | | | | | |
| 88. | Circular | | | | | |
| 89. | Spiral | | | | | |
| 90. | Reverse spiral | | | | | |
| 91. | Recurrent | | | | | |
| 92. | Spica | | | | | |
| 93. | Figure of eight | | | | | |
| 94. | Eye | | | | | |

| S. No. | Procedural competencies/ skill | Performs independently | Assist/observes procedure (A/O) | Date | | Signature of the tutor/ faculty |
|---|---|---|---|---|---|---|
| | | | | Skill lab/ simulation lab | Clinical area | |
| 95. | Ear | | | | | |
| 96. | Caplin | | | | | |
| 97. | Jaw | | | | | |
| 98. | Arm sling | | | | | |
| 99. | Abdominal binder | | | | | |
| 100. | Basic CPR (First aid module) | | | | | |

Signature of Class-coordinator

Date:

Signature of Principal with seal

Date:

## CLINICAL REQUIREMENTS

| S. No. | Clinical requirements | Date | Signature of faculty |
|---|---|---|---|
| 1. | History taking-2<br>1.<br>2. | | |
| 2. | Physical examination-2<br>1.<br>2. | | |
| 3. | Fall risk assessment-2<br>1.<br>2. | | |
| 4. | Pressure sore assessment-2<br>1.<br>2. | | |
| 5. | Nursing process-2<br>1.<br>2. | | |
| 6. | Completion of first aid module | | |
| 7. | Completion of health assessment module | | |

Signature of Class-coordinator

Date:

Signature of Principal with seal

Date:

## PRACTICAL EXAMINATION

**First Attempt**

Signature of Internal Examiner

Signature of External Examiner

Date:

Date:

**Second Attempt**

Signature of Internal Examiner

Signature of External Examiner

Date:

Date:

**Third Attempt**

Signature of Internal Examiner

Signature of External Examiner

Date:

Date:

**Fourth Attempt**

Signature of Internal Examiner

Signature of External Examiner

Date:

Date:

# SEMESTER –III: ADULT HEALTH NURSING-I

| S. No. | Procedural competencies/skill | Performs independently | Assist/observes procedure (A/O) | Date | | Signature of the tutor/ faculty |
|---|---|---|---|---|---|---|
| | | | | Skill lab/ simulation lab | Clinical area | |
| **I. Medical** | | | | | | |
| *A. Intravenous Therapy* | | | | | | |
| 1. | IV cannulation | | | | | |
| 2. | IV maintenance and monitoring | | | | | |
| 3. | Administration of IV medications | | | | | |
| 4. | Care of patient with central line | | | | | |
| *B. Preparation, assisting and after care of patients undergoing diagnostic procedures* | | | | | | |
| 5. | Thoracientesis | | | | | |
| 6. | Abdominal parencentesis | | | | | |
| *C. Respiratory therapies and monitoring* | | | | | | |
| 7. | Administration of oxygen using venture mask | | | | | |
| 8. | Nebulization | | | | | |
| 9. | Chest physiotherapy | | | | | |
| 10. | Postural drainage | | | | | |
| 11. | Oropharyngeal suctioning | | | | | |
| 12. | Care of patient with chest drainage | | | | | |
| *D. Planning therapeutic diet* | | | | | | |
| 13. | High protein | | | | | |
| 14. | Diabetic diet | | | | | |
| 15. | Performing and monitoring GRBS | | | | | |
| 16. | Insulin administration | | | | | |
| **II. Surgical** | | | | | | |
| 17. | Pre-operative care | | | | | |
| 18. | Immediate post-operative care | | | | | |
| 19. | Post-operative exercises | | | | | |
| 20. | Pain assessment and management | | | | | |
| *E. Assisting diagnostic procedures and after care of patients undergoing* | | | | | | |
| 21. | Colostomy | | | | | |
| 22. | ERCP | | | | | |
| 23. | Endoscopy | | | | | |
| 24. | Liver biopsy | | | | | |
| 25. | Nasogastric aspiration | | | | | |
| 26. | Gastroscopy/jejunoscopy | | | | | |
| 27. | Ileostomy/colostomy care | | | | | |
| 28. | Surgical dressing | | | | | |
| 29. | Suture removal | | | | | |
| 30. | Surgical soak | | | | | |
| 31. | Sitz bath | | | | | |
| 32. | Care of drain | | | | | |

| S. No. | Procedural competencies/skill | Performs independently | Assist/observes procedure (A/O) | Date | | Signature of the tutor/ faculty |
|---|---|---|---|---|---|---|
| | | | | Skill lab/ simulation lab | Clinical area | |
| **III. Cardiology** | | | | | | |
| 33. | Cardiac monitoring | | | | | |
| 34. | Recording and interpreting ECG | | | | | |
| 35. | Arterial blood gas analysis and interpretation | | | | | |
| 36. | Administration of cardiac drugs | | | | | |
| 37. | Preparation and after care of patients undergoing cardiac catheterization | | | | | |
| 38. | Performing BCLS | | | | | |
| *F. Collection of blood samples for* | | | | | | |
| 39. | Blood grouping/cross matching | | | | | |
| 40. | Blood sugar | | | | | |
| 41. | Serum electrolytes | | | | | |
| 42. | Assisting with blood transfusion | | | | | |
| 43. | Assisting for bone marrow aspiration | | | | | |
| 44. | Application of anti-embolism stocking (TED hose) | | | | | |
| 45. | Application/maintenance of sequential compression device | | | | | |
| **IV. Dermatology** | | | | | | |
| 46. | Application of topical medications | | | | | |
| 47. | Intradermal injection—skin allergy testing | | | | | |
| 48. | Medicated bath | | | | | |
| **V. Communicable** | | | | | | |
| 49. | Intradermal injection—BCG and tuberculosis skin test for Mantoux test | | | | | |
| 50. | Barrier nursing and reverse barrier nursing | | | | | |
| 51. | Standard precautions—hand hygiene, use of PPE, needle stick and sharp injury prevention, cleaning and disinfection, respiratory hygiene, waste disposal and safe injection practices | | | | | |
| **VI. Musculoskeletal** | | | | | | |
| 52. | Preparation of patient with myelogram/CT/MRI | | | | | |
| 53. | Assisting with application and removal of POP/cast | | | | | |
| 54. | Preparation, assisting and after care of patient with skin traction/skeletal traction | | | | | |
| 55. | Care of orthotics | | | | | |
| 56. | Muscle strengthening exercises | | | | | |

| S. No. | Procedural competencies/skill | Performs independently | Assist/observes procedure (A/O) | Date | | Signature of the tutor/ faculty |
|---|---|---|---|---|---|---|
| | | | | Skill lab/ simulation lab | Clinical area | |
| 57. | Crutch walking | | | | | |
| 58. | Rehabilitation | | | | | |
| **VII. On routine procedures** | | | | | | |
| 59. | Position and draping | | | | | |
| 60. | Preparation of operation table | | | | | |
| 61. | Set-up of trolley with instrument | | | | | |
| 62. | Assisting in major and minor operation | | | | | |
| 63. | Disinfection and sterilization of equipment | | | | | |
| 64. | Scrubbing procedures—gowning, masking and gloving | | | | | |
| 65. | Intraoperative monitoring | | | | | |

Signature of Class-coordinator

Date:

Signature of Principal with seal

Date:

**Internal Practical Examination of Nursing Foundation**

Signature of Examiner-I

Name:

Date:

Signature of Examiner-II

Name:

Date:

## CLINICAL REQUIREMENTS

| S. No. | Clinical requirements | Date | Signature of faculty |
|---|---|---|---|
| **A. Medical** | | | |
| 1. | Case study-1 | | |
| 2. | Health education-1 | | |
| 3. | Clinical presentation/care note-1 | | |
| **B. Surgical** | | | |
| 4. | Care study-1 | | |
| 5. | Health education-1 | | |
| 6. | Clinical presentation/care note-1 | | |
| **C. Cardiac** | | | |
| 7. | Cardiac assessment-1 | | |
| 8. | Drug presentation-1 | | |
| **D. Communicable** | | | |
| 9. | Clinical presentation/care note-1 | | |
| **E. Musculoskeletal** | | | |
| 10. | Clinical presentation/care note-1 | | |
| **F. On Routine procedures** | | | |
| 11. | Assist in circulatory nurse-5<br>1.<br>2.<br>3.<br>4.<br>5. | | |
| 12. | Assist as scrub nurse in minor surgeries-5<br>1.<br>2.<br>3.<br>4.<br>5. | | |
| 13. | Positioning and draping -5<br>1.<br>2.<br>3.<br>4.<br>5. | | |

| S. No. | Clinical requirements | Date | Signature of faculty |
|---|---|---|---|
| 14. | Assist as scrub nurse in major surgeries-5<br>1.<br>2.<br>3.<br>4.<br>5. | | |
| 15. | Completion of BCLS module | | |

Signature of Class-coordinator

Date:

Signature of Principal with seal

Date:

## PRACTICAL EXAMINATION

**First Attempt**

Signature of Internal Examiner | Signature of External Examiner

Date: | Date:

**Second Attempt**

Signature of Internal Examiner | Signature of External Examiner

Date: | Date:

**Third Attempt**

Signature of Internal Examiner | Signature of External Examiner

Date: | Date:

**Fourth Attempt**

Signature of Internal Examiner | Signature of External Examiner

Date: | Date:

## SEMESTER –IV: ADULT HEALTH NURSING-II

| S. No. | Procedural competencies/skill | Performs independently | Assist/observes procedure (A/O) | Date | | Signature of the tutor/ faculty |
|---|---|---|---|---|---|---|
| | | | | Skill lab/ simulation lab | Clinical area | |
| **I. ENT** | | | | | | |
| 1. | History taking and examination of ear, nose and throat | | | | | |
| 2. | Application of bandages to ear and nose | | | | | |
| 3. | Tracheostomy | | | | | |
| *A. Preparation of patient, assisting and monitoring of patients undergoing diagnostic tests* | | | | | | |
| 4. | Auditory screening tests | | | | | |
| 5. | Audiometric tests | | | | | |
| 6. | Preparing and assisting in special procedure like anterior/posterior nasal packing, ear packing and syringing | | | | | |
| 7. | Preparation and after care of patients undergoing ENT surgical procedures | | | | | |
| 8. | Instilling of ear/nasal medication | | | | | |
| **II. Eye** | | | | | | |
| 9. | History taking and examination of eyes and interpretation | | | | | |
| *B. Assisting procedure* | | | | | | |
| 10. | Visual acuity | | | | | |
| 11. | Fundoscopy, retinoscopy, opthalmoscopy, tonometry | | | | | |
| 12. | Refractory tests | | | | | |
| 13. | Pre and post-operative care of patient undergoing eye surgery | | | | | |
| 14. | Instillation of eye drops/medication | | | | | |
| 15. | Eye irrigation | | | | | |

| S. No. | Procedural competencies/skill | Performs independently | Assist/observes procedure (A/O) | Date | | Signature of the tutor/ faculty |
|---|---|---|---|---|---|---|
| | | | | Skill lab/ simulation lab | Clinical area | |
| 16. | Application of eye bandage | | | | | |
| 17. | Assisting with foreign body removal | | | | | |
| **III. Nephrology** | | | | | | |
| 18. | Assessment of kidney and urinary system:<br>a. History taking and physical examination | | | | | |
| 19. | Cystoscopy, cysrometrogram | | | | | |
| 20. | Contrast studies—IVP | | | | | |
| 21. | Peritoneal dialysis | | | | | |
| 22. | Hemodialysis | | | | | |
| 23. | Care of hemodialysis machine | | | | | |
| 24. | Renal/prostate biopsy | | | | | |
| 25. | Specific test—semen analysis, gonorrhea test | | | | | |
| 26. | Catheterization care | | | | | |
| 27. | Bladder irrigation | | | | | |
| 28. | Intake and output recording and monitoring | | | | | |
| 29. | Ambulation and exercise | | | | | |
| **IV. Burns and reconstruction surgery** | | | | | | |
| 30. | Assessment of burns wounds—area/degree/ percentage of wound using appropriate scale | | | | | |
| 31. | First aid for burns | | | | | |
| 32. | Fluid and electrolyte replacement therapy | | | | | |
| 33. | Skin care | | | | | |
| 34. | Care of burn wounds<br>a. Bathing<br>b. Dressing | | | | | |
| 35. | Pre-operative and post-operative care of patient with burns | | | | | |

| S. No. | Procedural competencies/skill | Performs independently | Assist/observes procedure (A/O) | Date | | Signature of the tutor/ faculty |
|---|---|---|---|---|---|---|
| | | | | Skill lab/ simulation lab | Clinical area | |
| 36. | Caring of skin graft and post-cosmetic surgery | | | | | |
| 37. | Rehabilitation | | | | | |
| **V. Neurology** | | | | | | |
| 38. | History taking, neurological examination—use of Glasgow Coma Scale | | | | | |
| 39. | Continuous monitoring the patient | | | | | |
| 40. | Preparation and assisting for various invasive and non-invasive diagnostic procedure | | | | | |
| 41. | Care of patient undergoing neurosurgery including rehabilitation | | | | | |
| **VI. Immunology** | | | | | | |
| 42. | History taking and physical examination | | | | | |
| 43. | Immunological status assessment and interpretation of specific test (e.g. HIV) | | | | | |
| 44. | Care of patient with low immunity | | | | | |
| **VII. Oncology** | | | | | | |
| 45. | History taking and physical examination of cancer patients | | | | | |
| 46. | Screening for common cancer—TNM classification | | | | | |
| *C. Preparation, assisting and after care patients undergoing diagnostic procedures* | | | | | | |
| 47. | Biopsies/FNAC | | | | | |
| 48. | Bone marrow aspiration | | | | | |
| *D. Preparation of patient and assisting with various modalities of treatment* | | | | | | |
| 49. | Chemotherapy | | | | | |
| 50. | Radiotherapy | | | | | |
| 51. | Hormonal therapy/ immunotherapy | | | | | |

| S. No. | Procedural competencies/skill | Performs independently | Assist/observes procedure (A/O) | Date | | Signature of the tutor/ faculty |
|---|---|---|---|---|---|---|
| | | | | Skill lab/ simulation lab | Clinical area | |
| 52. | Gene therapy/any other | | | | | |
| 53. | Care of patients treated with nuclear medicine | | | | | |
| 54. | Rehabilitation | | | | | |
| **VIII. Emergency** | | | | | | |
| 55. | Practicing triage | | | | | |
| 56. | Primary and secondary survey in emergency | | | | | |
| 57. | Examination, investigations and their interpretations in emergency and disaster situation | | | | | |
| 58. | Emergency care of medical and traumatic injury patients | | | | | |
| 59. | Documentation and assisting in legal procedures in emergency unit | | | | | |
| 60. | Managing crowd | | | | | |
| 61. | Counseling the patient and family in dealing with grieving and bereavement | | | | | |
| **IX. Critical care** | | | | | | |
| 62. | Assessment of critically ill patients | | | | | |
| 63. | Assisting with arterial puncture | | | | | |
| 64. | Assisting with ET tube intubation and extubation | | | | | |
| 65. | ABG analysis and interpretation—respiratory acidosis, respiratory alkalosis, metabolic acidosis, metabolic alkalosis | | | | | |
| 66. | Setting-up of ventilator modes and setting and care of patient on ventilator | | | | | |
| 67. | Setting up of trolley with instruments | | | | | |

| S. No. | Procedural competencies/skill | Performs independently | Assist/observes procedure (A/O) | Date | | Signature of the tutor/ faculty |
|---|---|---|---|---|---|---|
| | | | | Skill lab/ simulation lab | Clinical area | |
| 68. | Monitoring and maintenance of chest drainage system | | | | | |
| 69. | Bag and mask ventilation | | | | | |
| 70. | Assisting with starting and maintenance of central and pheripheral lines invasive | | | | | |
| 71. | Setting up infusion pump | | | | | |
| 72. | Administration of drugs via infusion, intra-cardiac, intra-thecal, epidural | | | | | |
| 73. | Monitoring and maintenance of pacemaker | | | | | |
| 74. | ICU care bundle | | | | | |
| 75. | Management of the dying patient in the ICU | | | | | |
| **X** | **Geriatric** | | | | | |
| 76. | History taking and assessment of geriatric patient | | | | | |
| 77. | Geriatric counseling | | | | | |
| 78. | Comprehensive health assessment (adult) after module completion | | | | | |

Signature of Class-coordinator

Date:

Signature of Principal with seal

Date:

**Internal Practical Examination of Nursing Foundation**

Signature of Examiner-I

Name:

Date:

Signature of Examiner-II

Name:

Date:

## CLINICAL REQUIREMENTS

| S. No. | Clinical requirements | Date | Signature of faculty |
|---|---|---|---|
| **A. ENT** | | | |
| 1. | ENT assessment of an adult<br>1.<br><br>2. | | |
| 2. | Observation and activity report of OPD | | |
| 3. | Clinical presentation-1 | | |
| 4. | Drug chart | | |
| **B. Eye** | | | |
| 5. | Eye assessment<br>1. Adult-1<br>2. Geriatric | | |
| 6. | Patient teaching-1 | | |
| 7. | Clinical presentation-1 | | |
| **C. Nephrology and urology** | | | |
| 8. | Assessment of adult-2<br>Assessment of geriatric-1 | | |
| 9. | Drug presentation-1 | | |
| | | | |
| 10. | Care study/clinical presentation-1 | | |
| **D. Burns and reconstructive surgery** | | | |
| 11. | Burns wound assessment | | |
| 12. | Clinical presentation-1 | | |
| 13. | Observation report of burns unit | | |
| 14. | Observe cosmetic/reconstructive procedures | | |
| **E. Nephrology** | | | |
| 15. | Neuro assessment-2<br>a.<br><br>b. | | |
| 16. | Unconscious patient-1 | | |
| 17. | Case study/case presentation-1 | | |
| 18. | Drug presentation-1 | | |
| **F. Immunology** | | | |
| 19. | Assessment of immune status | | |
| 20. | Teaching of isolation to patient and family care givers | | |
| 21. | Nutritional management | | |
| 22. | Care note-1 | | |
| **G. Oncology** | | | |
| 23. | Observation report of cancer unit | | |
| 24. | Assessment of each system cancer patients-2 | | |
| 25. | Care study/clinical presentation -1 | | |

| S. No. | Clinical requirements | Date | Signature of faculty |
|---|---|---|---|
| 26. | Pre and post-operative care of patient with various modes of cancer treatment such as chemotherapy, radiation therapy, surgery, BMT, etc—3 (at least)<br>a.<br>b.<br>c. | | |
| 27. | Teaching on BSE to family members | | |
| **H. Emergency** | | | |
| 28. | Primary assessment of adult-1 | | |
| 29. | Immediate care (IV access establishment, assisting in intubation, suction etc) | | |
| 30. | Use of emergency trolley | | |
| **I. Critical care** | | | |
| 31. | Assessment of critically ill<br>a.<br>b. | | |
| 32. | Care note/clinical presentation-1 | | |
| **J. Geriatric** | | | |
| 33. | Geriatric assessment -1 | | |
| 34. | Care note/clinical assessment | | |
| 35. | Fall risk assessment-1 | | |
| 36. | Functional status assessment -1 | | |
| 37. | Completion of fundamentals of prescribing module | | |
| 38. | Completion of palliative care module | | |

Signature of Class-coordinator

Date:

Signature of Principal with seal

Date:

## PRACTICAL EXAMINATION

**First Attempt**

Signature of Internal Examiner

Date:

Signature of External Examiner

Date:

**Second Attempt**

Signature of Internal Examiner

Date:

Signature of External Examiner

Date:

**Third Attempt**

Signature of Internal Examiner

Date:

Signature of External Examiner

Date:

**Fourth Attempt**

Signature of Internal Examiner

Date:

Signature of External Examiner

Date:

# SEMESTER –V: EDUCATIONAL TECHNOLOGY/NURSING EDUCATION

| S. No. | Procedural competencies/ skill | Performs independently | Assist/ observes procedure (A/O) | Date | | Signature of the tutor/ faculty |
|---|---|---|---|---|---|---|
| | | | | Skill lab/simulation lab | Clinical area | |
| 1. | Writing learning outcomes | | | | | |
| 2. | Preparation of lesson plan | | | | | |
| 3. | Practice teaching/ microteaching | | | | | |
| 4. | Preparation of teaching aids/medias | | | | | |
| **A. Preparation of assessment tools** | | | | | | |
| 5. | Construction of MCQs | | | | | |
| 6. | Preparation of observation checklist | | | | | |

## CLINICAL REQUIREMENTS

| S. No. | Clinical requirements | Date | Signature of faculty |
|---|---|---|---|
| 1. | Microteaching -2<br>a. Theory-1<br>b. Practical/lab-1 | | |
| 2. | Field visit to nursing educational institution-regional/national organization<br>a.<br>b.<br>c. | | |

Signature of Class-coordinator

Date:

Signature of Principal with seal

Date:

## COMMUNITY HEALTH NURSING-I INCLUDING ENVIRONMENTAL SCIENCES AND EPIDEMIOLOGY

| S. No. | Procedural competencies/skill | Performs independently | Assist/ observes procedure (A/O) | Date | | Signature of the tutor/ faculty |
|---|---|---|---|---|---|---|
| | | | | Skill lab/ simulation lab | Clinical area | |
| 1. | Interviewing skills (using communication and interpersonal skills) | | | | | |
| 2. | Conducting community needs assessment/survey | | | | | |
| 3. | Observation skills | | | | | |
| 4. | Nutritional assessment skills | | | | | |
| 5. | Teaching individuals and families on nutrition-food hygiene and safety, healthy life style and health promotion | | | | | |
| 6. | BCC (Behavior change communication) skills | | | | | |
| 7. | Health assessment including nutritional assessment—different age groups<br>a. Children under five<br>b. Adolescent<br>c. Women | | | | | |
| 8. | Investing an epidemic community health survey | | | | | |
| 9. | Performing lab tests—hemoglobin, blood sugar, blood smear for malaria, etc. | | | | | |
| 10. | Screening, diagnosis and primary management of common health problems in the community and referral of high risk clients (communicable and NCD) | | | | | |
| 11. | Documentation skills | | | | | |
| 12. | Home visit | | | | | |
| 13. | Participation in national health programmes | | | | | |
| 14. | Participation in school health program | | | | | |

Signature of Class-coordinator

Date:

Signature of Principal with seal

Date:

## CLINICAL REQUIREMENTS

| S. No. | Clinical requirements | Date | Signature of faculty |
|---|---|---|---|
| 1. | Community needs assessment/survey (Rural/urban) -1 | | |
| 2. | Visits to<br>SC/HWC<br>PHC<br>CHC | | |
| 3. | Observation of nutritional programs<br>Anganwadi | | |
| 4. | Observational visits<br>1. Water purification site and water quality tests<br>2. Milk dairy<br>3. Slaughter house<br>4. Market<br>5. Sewage disposal site<br>6. Rain water harvesting | | |
| 5. | Nutritional assessment—adult-1 | | |
| 6. | Individual health teaching—adult-1 | | |
| 7. | Use of AV aids—flash cards/posters/flannel graphs/flip charts (any two)<br>a.<br>b. | | |
| 8. | Health assessment of<br>1. Women-1<br>2. Infant/under five child-1<br>3. Adolescent-1<br>4. Adult-1 | | |
| 9. | Growth monitoring of children under five-1 | | |
| 10. | Documentation<br>1. Individual record<br>2. Family records | | |
| 11. | Investigating of epidemic-1 | | |
| 12. | Screening and primary management of<br>1. Communicable diseases<br>2. NCD-1 | | |
| 13. | Home visits-2 | | |
| 14. | Participation in national health program-1 | | |
| 15. | Participation in school health program-2 | | |

Signature of Class-coordinator

Date:

Signature of Principal with seal

Date:

## PRACTICAL EXAMINATION

**First Attempt**

Signature of Internal Examiner

Date:

Signature of External Examiner

Date:

**Second Attempt**

Signature of Internal Examiner

Date:

Signature of External Examiner

Date:

**Third Attempt**

Signature of Internal Examiner

Date:

Signature of External Examiner

Date:

**Fourth Attempt**

Signature of Internal Examiner

Date:

Signature of External Examiner

Date:

## SEMESTER –V AND VI: CHILD HEALTH NURSING-I AND II

| S. No. | Procedural competencies/skill | Performs independently | Assist/ observes procedure (A/O) | Date | | Signature of the tutor/ faculty |
|---|---|---|---|---|---|---|
| | | | | Skill lab/ simulation lab | Clinical area | |
| **I. Pediatric medical and surgical** | | | | | | |
| *A. Health assessment—taking history and physical examination and nutritional assessment* | | | | | | |
| 1. | Neonate | | | | | |
| 2. | Infant | | | | | |
| 3. | Toddler | | | | | |
| 4. | Preschooler | | | | | |
| 5. | Schooler | | | | | |
| 6. | Adolescent | | | | | |
| *B. Assessment of medications/fluids—calculation, preparation and administration of medications* | | | | | | |
| 7. | Oral | | | | | |
| 8. | IM | | | | | |
| 9. | IV | | | | | |
| 10. | Intramuscular | | | | | |
| 11. | Subcutaneous | | | | | |
| 12. | Calculation of fluid requirements | | | | | |
| 13. | Preparation of different strengths of IV fluids | | | | | |
| 14. | Administration of IV fluids | | | | | |
| 15. | Applications of restraints | | | | | |
| *C. Administration of $O_2$ inhalation by different methods* | | | | | | |
| 16. | Nasal catheter/nasal prong | | | | | |
| 17. | Mask | | | | | |
| 18. | Oxygen hood | | | | | |
| 19. | Baby bath/sponge bath | | | | | |
| 20. | Feeding children by katori and spoon/ paladai, cup | | | | | |
| *D. Collection of specimen for common investigation* | | | | | | |
| 21. | Urine | | | | | |
| 22. | Stool | | | | | |
| 23. | Blood | | | | | |

| S. No. | Procedural competencies/skill | Performs independently | Assist/ observes procedure (A/O) | Date | | Signature of the tutor/ faculty |
|---|---|---|---|---|---|---|
| | | | | Skill lab/ simulation lab | Clinical area | |
| 24. | Assisting with common diagnostic procedures (lumbar puncture, bone marrow aspiration) | | | | | |
| *E. Health education to mother/parents-topics* | | | | | | |
| 25. | Prevention and management of malnutrition | | | | | |
| 26. | Prevention and management of diarrhea (oral rehydration therapy) | | | | | |
| 27. | Feeding and complementary feeding | | | | | |
| 28. | Immunization schedule | | | | | |
| 29. | Play therapy | | | | | |
| 30. | Conduct individual and group play therapy sessions | | | | | |
| 31. | Prevention of accidents | | | | | |
| 32. | Bowel wash | | | | | |
| 33. | Administration of suppositories | | | | | |
| *F. Care of ostomies* | | | | | | |
| 34. | Colostomy irrigations | | | | | |
| 35. | Ureterostomy | | | | | |
| 36. | Gastrostomy | | | | | |
| 37. | Enterostomy | | | | | |
| 38. | Urinary catheterization and drainage | | | | | |
| *G.* | *Feeding* | | | | | |
| 39. | Nasogastric | | | | | |
| 40. | Gastrostomy | | | | | |
| 41. | Jejunostomy | | | | | |
| *H. Care of surgical wounds* | | | | | | |
| 42. | Dressing | | | | | |
| 43. | Suture removal | | | | | |

| S. No. | Procedural competencies/skill | Performs independently | Assist/ observes procedure (A/O) | Date | | Signature of the tutor/ faculty |
|---|---|---|---|---|---|---|
| | | | | Skill lab/ simulation lab | Clinical area | |
| **II. Pediatric OPD/imminization room** | | | | | | |
| *I. Pediatric and developmental assessment of children* | | | | | | |
| 44. | Infant | | | | | |
| 45. | Toddler | | | | | |
| 46. | Preschooler | | | | | |
| 47. | Schooler | | | | | |
| 48. | Adolescent | | | | | |
| 49. | Administration of vaccination | | | | | |
| 50. | Health/nutritional status | | | | | |
| **III. NICU/PICU** | | | | | | |
| 51. | Assessment of newborn | | | | | |
| 52. | Care of preterm/LBW newborn | | | | | |
| 53. | Kangaroo care | | | | | |
| 54. | Neonatal resuscitation | | | | | |
| 55. | Assisting in neonatal diagnostic procedures | | | | | |
| 56. | Feeding of highrisk newborn—EBM (spoon/paladin) | | | | | |
| 57. | Insertion/removal/ feeding- naso/oral-gastric tubes | | | | | |
| 58. | Administration of medication-oral/ parentral | | | | | |
| 59. | Neonatal drug calculation | | | | | |
| 60. | Assisting in exchange transfusion | | | | | |
| 61. | Organizing different levels of neonatal care | | | | | |
| 62. | Care of a child on ventilator CPAP | | | | | |
| 63. | Endotracheal suction | | | | | |
| 64. | Chest physiotherapy | | | | | |
| 65. | Administration of fluids with infusion pumps | | | | | |

| S. No. | Procedural competencies/skill | Performs independently | Assist/ observes procedure (A/O) | Date | | Signature of the tutor/ faculty |
|---|---|---|---|---|---|---|
| | | | | Skill lab/ simulation lab | Clinical area | |
| 66. | Total parental nutrition | | | | | |
| 67. | Recording and reporting | | | | | |
| 68. | Cardiopulmonary resuscitation-PLS | | | | | |

## CLINICAL REQUIREMENTS

| S. No. | Clinical requirements | Date | Signature of faculty |
|---|---|---|---|
| **A. Pediatric medical** | | | |
| 1. | Nursing care plan-1 | | |
| 2. | Case presentation-1 | | |
| 3. | Health talk-1 | | |
| **B. Surgical** | | | |
| 4. | Nursing care plan-1 | | |
| 5. | Case study presentation-1 | | |
| **C. OPD/Immunization room** | | | |
| 6. | Growth and development study<br>a. Infant-1<br>b. Toddler-1<br>c. Preschooler-1 | | |
| **D. NICCU/PICU** | | | |
| 7. | Newborn assessment-1 | | |
| 8. | Nursing care plan-1 | | |
| 9. | Kangaroo mother care-2 | | |
| 10. | Nursing care plan of high risk newborn-1 | | |
| 11. | Completion of ENBC Module | | |
| 12. | Completion of FNBC Module | | |
| 13. | Completion of IMNCI Module | | |
| 14. | Completion of PLS Module | | |

Signature of Class-coordinator

Date:

Signature of Principal with seal

Date:

## SEMESTER –V AND VI: MENTAL HEALTH NURSING-I AND II

| S. No. | Procedural competencies/skill | Performs independently | Assist/observes procedure (A/O) | Date | | Signature of the tutor/ faculty |
|---|---|---|---|---|---|---|
| | | | | Skill lab/ simulation lab | Clinical area | |
| **I. Psychiatric OPD** | | | | | | |
| 1. | History taking | | | | | |
| 2. | Mental status examination | | | | | |
| 3. | Psychometric assessment (observer/ practice) | | | | | |
| 4. | Neurological examination | | | | | |
| 5. | Observing and assisting in therapies | | | | | |
| *A. Individual and group psycho education* | | | | | | |
| 6. | Mental health practice education | | | | | |
| 7. | Family psycho-education | | | | | |
| **II. Child guidance clinic** | | | | | | |
| 8. | History taking and mental status examination | | | | | |
| 9. | Psychometric assessment (observe/ practice) | | | | | |
| 10. | Observing and assisting in various therapies | | | | | |
| 11. | Parental teaching for child with mental deficiencies | | | | | |
| **III. In-patient ward** | | | | | | |
| 12. | History taking | | | | | |
| 13. | Mental status examination (MSE) | | | | | |
| 14. | Neurological examination | | | | | |
| 15. | Assisting in psychometric assessment | | | | | |
| 16. | Recording therapeutic communication | | | | | |
| 17. | Administration of medications | | | | | |

| S. No. | Procedural competencies/skill | Performs independently | Assist/observes procedure (A/O) | Date | | Signature of the tutor/ faculty |
|---|---|---|---|---|---|---|
| | | | | Skill lab/ simulation lab | Clinical area | |
| 18. | Assisting in electroconvulsive therapy (ECT) | | | | | |
| 19. | Participation in all therapies | | | | | |
| 20. | Prepare of patients for activities of daily living (ADLs) | | | | | |
| 21. | Conducting admission and discharge counseling | | | | | |
| 22. | Counseling and teaching patients and families | | | | | |
| **IV. Community psychiatry and de-addictive center** | | | | | | |
| 23. | Conducting home visit and case work | | | | | |
| 24. | Identification of individuals with mental health problems | | | | | |
| 25. | Assisting in organization of mental health camp | | | | | |
| 26. | Conducting awareness meeting for mental health and mental illness | | | | | |
| 27. | Counseling and teaching family members, parents and community | | | | | |
| 28. | Observation of de-addiction care | | | | | |

Signature of Class-coordinator

Date:

Signature of Principal with seal

Date:

## CLINICAL REQUIREMENTS

| S. No. | Clinical requirements | Date | Signature of faculty |
|---|---|---|---|
| **A. Psychiatric OPD** | | | |
| 1. | History taking and mental status examination-2<br>a.<br>b. | | |
| 2. | Health education-1 | | |
| 3. | Observation report of OPD | | |
| **B. Child guidance clinic** | | | |
| 4. | Care work-1 | | |
| **C. In-patient ward** | | | |
| 5. | Case study-1 | | |
| 6. | Care plan-2 | | |
| 7. | Clinical presentation-1 | | |
| 8. | Process recording-2 | | |
| 9. | Maintain drug book | | |
| **D. Community psychiatric and de-addiction center** | | | |
| 10. | Case work-1 | | |
| 11. | Observation report on field visits | | |
| 12. | Visits to de-addication center | | |

Signature of Class-coordinator

Date:

Signature of Principal with seal

Date:

# SEMESTER –V AND VI: CHILD HEALTH NURSING-I AND II

## PRACTICAL EXAMINATION

**First Attempt**

Signature of Internal Examiner

Signature of External Examiner

Date:

Date:

**Second Attempt**

Signature of Internal Examiner

Signature of External Examiner

Date:

Date:

**Third Attempt**

Signature of Internal Examiner

Signature of External Examiner

Date:

Date:

**Fourth Attempt**

Signature of Internal Examiner

Signature of External Examiner

Date:

Date:

# SEMESTER –V AND VI: MENTAL HEALTH NURSING-I AND II

## PRACTICAL EXAMINATION

**First Attempt**

Signature of Internal Examiner | Signature of External Examiner

Date: | Date:

**Second Attempt**

Signature of Internal Examiner | Signature of External Examiner

Date: | Date:

**Third Attempt**

Signature of Internal Examiner | Signature of External Examiner

Date: | Date:

**Fourth Attempt**

Signature of Internal Examiner | Signature of External Examiner

Date: | Date:

# SEMESTER –VI: NURSING MANAGEMENT AND LEADERSHIP

| S. No. | Procedural competencies/skill | Performs independently | Assist/observes procedure (A/O) | Date | | Signature of the tutor/ faculty |
|---|---|---|---|---|---|---|
| | | | | Skill lab/ simulation lab | Clinical area | |
| **I. Hospital and nursing service department** | | | | | | |
| 1. | Preparation of organogram (hospital/nursing department) | | | | | |
| 2. | Calculation of staffing requirements for a nursing unit/ward | | | | | |
| 3. | Formulation of job description of nursing officers (Staff nurse) | | | | | |
| 4. | Preparation of patient assignment plan | | | | | |
| 5. | Preparation of duty roster for staff/ students at different levels | | | | | |
| 6. | Preparation of log book/MMF for specific equipment/materials | | | | | |
| 7. | Participation in inventory control and daily record keeping | | | | | |
| 8. | Preparation and maintenance and reports such as incident report/ adverse reports/audit reports | | | | | |
| 9. | Participation in performance appraisal/evaluation of nursing personal | | | | | |
| 10. | Participate in conducting in-service education for the staff | | | | | |
| **II. College and hostel** | | | | | | |
| 11. | Preparation of organogram | | | | | |
| 12. | Formulation of job description for tutor | | | | | |
| 13. | Participation in performance appraisal of tutor | | | | | |
| 14. | Preparation of master plan, time-table and clinical rotation | | | | | |
| 15. | Preparation of student anecdotes | | | | | |
| 16. | Participation in clinical evaluation of students | | | | | |
| 17. | Participation in planning and conducting practical examination OSCE—end of posting | | | | | |

## CLINICAL REQUIREMENTS

| S. No. | Clinical requirements | Date | Signature of faculty |
|---|---|---|---|
| 1. | Field visit to hospital—regional/national organization | | |

Signature of Class-coordinator

Date:

Signature of Principal with seal

Date:

# SEMESTER –VI AND VII: MIDWIFERY/OBSTETRICS AND GYNECOLOGICAL (OBG) NURSING-I AND II

| S. No. | Procedural competencies/skill | Performs independently | Assist/ observes procedure (A/O) | Date | | Signature of the tutor/ faculty |
|---|---|---|---|---|---|---|
| | | | | Skill lab/ simulation lab | Clinical area | |
| **I. Antenatal care** | | | | | | |
| *A. Health assessment of antenatal women* | | | | | | |
| 1. | History taking including obstetrical score, calculation of EED, gestational age | | | | | |
| 2. | Physical examination—head to foot | | | | | |
| 3. | Obstetrical examination including leopards maneuvers and auscultation of fetal heart sound (fetoscope/stethoscope/Doppler) | | | | | |
| *B. Diagnostic tests* | | | | | | |
| 4. | Urine pregnancy test/card test | | | | | |
| 5. | Of hemoglobin using Sahli's hemoglobin meter | | | | | |
| 6. | Advice/assist in HIV/ HBsAg/VDRL testing | | | | | |
| 7. | Preparation of peripheral smear for malaria | | | | | |
| 8. | Urine testing for albumin and sugar | | | | | |
| 9. | Preparation of mother for USG | | | | | |
| 10. | Kick chart/DFMC (daily fetal and maternal chart) | | | | | |
| 11. | Preparation and recording of CTG/ NST | | | | | |
| 12. | Antenatal counseling for each trimester including birth preparedness | | | | | |
| 13. | Childbirth preparation classes for couples/family | | | | | |
| 14. | Administration of Td/TT | | | | | |
| 15. | Prescription of iron and folic acid and calcium tables | | | | | |
| **II. Intranatal Care** | | | | | | |
| 16. | Identification and assessment of women in labour | | | | | |
| 17. | Admission of women in labour | | | | | |
| 18. | Performing/assisting CTG | | | | | |

| S. No. | Procedural competencies/skill | Performs independently | Assist/ observes procedure (A/O) | Date | | Signature of the tutor/ faculty |
|---|---|---|---|---|---|---|
| | | | | Skill lab/ simulation lab | Clinical area | |
| 19. | Vaginal examination during labor including clinical pelvimetry | | | | | |
| 20. | Plotting and interpretation of partograph | | | | | |
| 21. | Preparation of birthing/delivery-physical and psychological | | | | | |
| 22. | Setting up of the birthing room/ delivery unit and newborn corner/ care area | | | | | |
| 23. | Pain management during labour-non-pharmacological | | | | | |
| 24. | Supporting normal births/conduct normal childbirth in upright position/evidence based | | | | | |
| 25. | Essential newborn care | | | | | |
| 26. | Basic newborn resuscitation | | | | | |
| 27. | Management of third stage of labour-physiologic management/ active management (AMTSL) | | | | | |
| 28. | Examination of placenta | | | | | |
| 29. | Care during fourth stage of labor | | | | | |
| 30. | Initiation of breast feeding and lactation management | | | | | |
| 31. | Infection prevention during labour and newborn care | | | | | |
| **III. Postnatal care** | | | | | | |
| 32. | Postnatal assessment and care | | | | | |
| 33. | Perineal/episiotomy care | | | | | |
| 34. | Breast care | | | | | |
| 35. | Postnatal counseling-diet, exercise and breast feeding | | | | | |
| 36. | Preparation for discharge | | | | | |
| **IV. Newborn care** | | | | | | |
| 37. | Assessment of newborn | | | | | |
| 38. | Weighing of newborn | | | | | |
| 39. | Administration of vitamin-K | | | | | |
| 40. | Neonatal immunization-administration of BCG, hepatitis B vaccine | | | | | |
| 41. | Identification of minor disorders of newborn and their management | | | | | |

| S. No. | Procedural competencies/skill | Performs independently | Assist/ observes procedure (A/O) | Date | | Signature of the tutor/ faculty |
|---|---|---|---|---|---|---|
| | | | | Skill lab/ simulation lab | Clinical area | |
| **V. Care of women with antenatal, intranatal and postnatal complications** | | | | | | |
| 42. | High-risk assessment-identification of antenatal complications such as pre-eclampsia, anemia, GDM, antepartum hemorrhage etc | | | | | |
| 43. | Post abortion care and counseling | | | | | |
| 44. | Glucose challenge test/glucose tolerance test | | | | | |
| 45. | Identification of fetal distress and its management | | | | | |
| 46. | Administration of $MgSO_4$ | | | | | |
| 47. | Administration of antenatal corticosteroids for preterm labour | | | | | |
| 48. | Assisting with medical induction of labour | | | | | |
| 49. | Assist in surgical induction-stripping and artificial rupture of membranes | | | | | |
| 50. | Episiotomy (only if required) and repair | | | | | |
| 51. | Preparation for emergency/elective cesarean section | | | | | |
| 52. | Assisting in cesarean section | | | | | |
| 53. | Preparation of mother and assist in vacuum delivery | | | | | |
| 54. | Identification and assisting in management of mal-presentation and mal-position during labour | | | | | |
| 55. | Preparation and assisting in low-forceps operation | | | | | |
| 56. | Preparation and assisting in emergency obstetric surgeries | | | | | |
| 57. | Prescription/administration of fluids and electrolytes through intravenous route | | | | | |
| **VI. Assisting in procedures** | | | | | | |
| 58. | Assisting in manual removal of the placenta | | | | | |
| 59. | Assisting in bimanual compression of uterus/balloon tamponade for Atonic uterus | | | | | |
| 60. | Assisting in aortic compression for PPH | | | | | |

| S. No. | Procedural competencies/skill | Performs independently | Assist/ observes procedure (A/O) | Date | | Signature of the tutor/ faculty |
|---|---|---|---|---|---|---|
| | | | | Skill lab/ simulation lab | Clinical area | |
| 61. | Identification and first aid management of PPH and obstetric shock | | | | | |
| 62. | Assisting in management of obstetric shock | | | | | |
| 63. | Identification and assisting in management of puerperal sepsis and administration of antibiotics | | | | | |
| 64. | Management of breast engorgement and infections | | | | | |
| 65. | Management of Thrombophlebitis | | | | | |
| 66. | Identification of high-risk newborn | | | | | |
| 67. | Care of neonate under radiant warmer | | | | | |
| 68. | Care of neonate on phototherapy | | | | | |
| 69. | Referral and transportation of high risk newborn | | | | | |
| 70. | Parental counseling-sick neonate and neonatal loss | | | | | |
| **VIII. Family welfare** | | | | | | |
| 71. | Postpartum family planning | | | | | |
| 72. | Postpartum family planning-insertion and removal of PPIUCD/ PAIUCD | | | | | |
| 73. | Counseling of the women for postpartum sterilization | | | | | |
| 74. | Preparation and assisting in tubectomy | | | | | |
| **IX** | **Other procedures** | | | | | |
| 75. | Preparation and assisting for D & C/D &E operations | | | | | |
| 76. | Observation/assisting in manual vacuum aspiration | | | | | |
| 77. | Assessment of women with gynecological disorders | | | | | |
| 78. | Assisting/performing pap smear | | | | | |
| 79. | Performing visual inspection of cervix with acetic acid | | | | | |
| 80. | Assisting/observation of cervical punch biopsy/cystoscopy/ cryosurgery | | | | | |
| 81. | Assisting in gynecological surgeries | | | | | |

| S. No. | Procedural competencies/skill | Performs independently | Assist/ observes procedure (A/O) | Date | | Signature of the tutor/ faculty |
|---|---|---|---|---|---|---|
| | | | | Skill lab/ simulation lab | Clinical area | |
| 82. | Postoperative care of women with gynecological surgeries | | | | | |
| 83. | Counsel on breast self-examination | | | | | |
| 84. | Counseling couples with infertility | | | | | |
| 85. | Competition of safe delivery app with certification | | | | | |

Signature of Class-coordinator

Date:

Signature of Principal with seal

Date:

**Internal Practical Examination of Nursing Foundation**

Signature of Examiner-I

Name:

Date:

Signature of Examiner-II

Name:

Date:

## CLINICAL REQUIREMENTS

| S. No. | Clinical requirements | Date | Signature of faculty |
|---|---|---|---|
| 1. | Antenatal assessment-20 | | |
| 2. | Postnatal assessment-15 | | |
| 3. | Assessment of labour using partograph-10 | | |
| 4. | Per vaginal examination-10 | | |
| 5. | Observing normal childbirths/deliveries-10 | | |
| 6. | Assisting in conduction of normal childbirth-10 | | |
| 7. | Conduction of normal deliveries-10 | | |
| 8. | Assisting in abnormal/institutional deliveries-5 | | |
| 9. | Performing placental examination-5 | | |
| 10. | Episiotomy and suturing (only if indicated)-3 | | |
| 11. | Assist/observe insertion of PPIUCD-2 | | |
| 12. | Newborn assessment-10 | | |
| 13. | Newborn resuscitation-5 | | |
| 14. | Kangaroo mother care-2 | | |
| | Nursing care plan/clinical presentation with drug study | | |
| 15. | Antenatal care<br>Normal (care plan)-1<br>High risk (clinical presentation)-1 | | |
| 16. | Intrapartum care<br>High-risk (clinical presentation)-1 | | |
| 17. | Postnatal care<br>Normal (care plan)-1<br>High risk (clinical presentation)-1<br>Newborn care<br>Normal (care plan)-1 | | |
| 18. | Gynecological condition<br>Care plan-1 | | |
| 19. | Health talk<br>Individual-1<br>Group-1 | | |
| 20. | Counseling mothers and family members | | |
| 21. | Visit to:<br>Peripheral health facility/laqshya certified labour room<br>Infertility center (virtual/videos) | | |
| 22. | Completion of SBA module | | |
| 23. | Completion of safe delivery app | | |

Signature of Class-coordinator

Date:

Signature of Principal with seal

Date:

# SEMESTER –VI AND VII: MIDWIFERY/OBSTETRICS AND GYNECOLOGICAL (OBG) NURSING-I AND II

## PRACTICAL EXAMINATION

**First Attempt**

Signature of Internal Examiner

Signature of External Examiner

Date:

Date:

**Second Attempt**

Signature of Internal Examiner

Signature of External Examiner

Date:

Date:

**Third Attempt**

Signature of Internal Examiner

Signature of External Examiner

Date:

Date:

**Fourth Attempt**

Signature of Internal Examiner

Signature of External Examiner

Date:

Date:

# SEMESTER –VII: NURSING RESEARCH AND STATISTICS

| S. No. | Procedural competencies/skill | Performs independently | Assist/ observes procedure (A/O) | Date | | Signature of the tutor/ faculty |
|---|---|---|---|---|---|---|
| | | | | Skill lab/ simulation lab | Clinical area | |
| **I. Research process exercise** | | | | | | |
| 1. | Statement of problem | | | | | |
| 2. | Formulation of objectives and hypothesis | | | | | |
| 3. | Literature review of research report/article | | | | | |
| 4. | Annotated bibliography | | | | | |
| 5. | Preparation of sample research tool | | | | | |
| **II. Analysis and interpretation of data—descriptive statistics** | | | | | | |
| 6. | Organization of data | | | | | |
| 7. | Tabulation of data | | | | | |
| 8. | Graphic representation of data | | | | | |
| 9. | Tabular presentation of data | | | | | |
| 10. | Research project (group/individual )<br>Title: | | | | | |

## CLINICAL REQUIREMENTS

| S. No. | Clinical requirements | Date | Signature of faculty |
|---|---|---|---|
| | Research project—group/individual<br>Title: | | |

Signature of Class-coordinator

Date:

Signature of Principal with seal

Date:

# COMMUNITY HEALTH NURSING-II

| S. No. | Procedural competencies/skill | Performs independently | Assist/ observes procedure (A/O) | Date | | Signature of the tutor/ faculty |
|---|---|---|---|---|---|---|
| | | | | Skill lab/ simulation lab | Clinical area | |
| 1. | Screening, diagnosing, management and referral of clients with common conditions/emergencies | | | | | |
| 2. | Antenatal and postnatal care and health center | | | | | |
| 3. | Conduction of normal childbirth and newborn care at health center | | | | | |
| 4. | Tracking every pregnancy and filling up MCP card | | | | | |
| 5. | Maintenance of records/registers/ reports | | | | | |
| 6. | Adolescent counseling and participation in youth friendly services | | | | | |
| 7. | Counseling for safe abortion services | | | | | |
| 8. | Family planning counseling | | | | | |
| 9. | Distribution of temporary contraceptives-condom's, OCP's, emergency contraceptives. Injectable MPA | | | | | |
| 10. | Insertion of interval IUCD | | | | | |
| 11. | Removal of IUCD | | | | | |
| 12. | Participation in conducting vasectomy/tubectomy camps | | | | | |
| 13. | Screening, diagnosis primary management and referral of clients with occupational health problems | | | | | |
| 14. | Health assessment of elderly | | | | | |
| 15. | Mental health screening | | | | | |
| 16. | Participating in community diagnosis-data management | | | | | |
| 17. | Writing health center activity report | | | | | |
| 18. | Participating in organizing and conducting clinical/health camp | | | | | |
| 19. | Participation in disaster mock drills | | | | | |
| 20. | Co-ordinating with ASHAs and other community health workers | | | | | |

## CLINICAL REQUIREMENTS

| S. No. | Clinical requirements | Date | Signature of faculty |
|---|---|---|---|
| 1. | Screening and primary management<br>a. Minor aliments -2<br>b. Emergencies-1<br>c. Dental problems-1<br>d. Eye-1<br>e. ENT-1 | | |
| 2. | Primary management and care based on protocols approved by MOH & FW (home/ health center) | | |
| 3. | Screening and primary management of:<br>a. Highrisk pregnancies<br>b. Highrisk neonate | | |
| 4. | Assessment of:<br>a. Antenatal-1<br>b. Intranatal-1<br>c. Postnatal-1<br>d. Newborn-1 | | |
| 5. | Conduction of normal childbirth and documentation-2 | | |
| 6. | Immediate newborn care and documentation | | |
| 7. | Family planning counseling-1 | | |
| 8. | Group health education (rural/urban) | | |
| 9. | Adolescent counseling -1 | | |
| 10. | Family case study (rural/urban) | | |
| 11. | Screening, diagnosis, primary management and referral of clients with occupational health problems-2<br>a.<br>b. | | |
| 12. | Health assessment (physical and nutritional) of elderly-1 | | |
| 13. | Mental health screening survey | | |
| 14. | Group project—community diagnosis (data management) | | |
| 15. | Writing report on health center activity | | |
| 16. | Participation in organizing and conducting under five/antenatal clinic/health camp<br>a.<br>b. | | |
| 17. | Participation in disaster mock drill | | |
| 18. | Field visits:<br>a. Biomedical waste management<br>b. AYUSH center<br>c. Industry<br>d. Geriatric home | | |
| 19. | Report on interaction with MPHW/HV/ASHA/AWWs (any two)<br>a.<br>b. | | |

Signature of Class-coordinator

Date:

Signature of Principal with seal

Date:

# COMMUNITY HEALTH NURSING-II

## PRACTICAL EXAMINATION

**First Attempt**

Signature of Internal Examiner

Signature of External Examiner

Date:

Date:

**Second Attempt**

Signature of Internal Examiner

Signature of External Examiner

Date:

Date:

**Third Attempt**

Signature of Internal Examiner

Signature of External Examiner

Date:

Date:

**Fourth Attempt**

Signature of Internal Examiner

Signature of External Examiner

Date:

Date:

# SEMESTER-VIII: INTERNSHIP CLINICAL REQUIREMENTS

| S. No. | Specialty | Area of posting | No. of days posting | Date | | Signature of the tutor/faculty |
|---|---|---|---|---|---|---|
| | | | | From | To | |
| 1. | Medical surgical nursing | | | | | |
| | | | | | | |
| | | | | | | |
| | | | | | | |
| | | | | | | |
| | | | | | | |
| | | | | | | |
| | | | | | | |
| 2. | Community health nursing | | | | | |
| | | | | | | |
| | | | | | | |
| | | | | | | |
| | | | | | | |
| | | | | | | |
| | | | | | | |
| | | | | | | |
| 3. | Child health nursing | | | | | |
| | | | | | | |
| | | | | | | |
| | | | | | | |
| | | | | | | |
| | | | | | | |
| | | | | | | |
| | | | | | | |
| 4. | OBG nursing | | | | | |
| | | | | | | |
| | | | | | | |
| | | | | | | |
| | | | | | | |
| | | | | | | |
| | | | | | | |
| | | | | | | |
| 5. | Mental health nursing | | | | | |
| | | | | | | |
| | | | | | | |
| | | | | | | |

Signature of Class-coordinator

Date:

Signature of Principal with seal

Date: